Adlin Alvelo Chacón
Yadira Hernández Sosa
Addinay Trujillo Rodríguez

Oral mucosal lesions

Adlin Alvelo Chacón
Yadira Hernández Sosa
Addinay Trujillo Rodríguez

Oral mucosal lesions

Study in Older Adults with removable dentures

ScienciaScripts

Imprint
Any brand names and product names mentioned in this book are subject to trademark, brand or patent protection and are trademarks or registered trademarks of their respective holders. The use of brand names, product names, common names, trade names, product descriptions etc. even without a particular marking in this work is in no way to be construed to mean that such names may be regarded as unrestricted in respect of trademark and brand protection legislation and could thus be used by anyone.

Cover image: www.ingimage.com

This book is a translation from the original published under ISBN 978-613-9-46593-4.

Publisher:
Sciencia Scripts
is a trademark of
Dodo Books Indian Ocean Ltd. and OmniScriptum S.R.L publishing group

120 High Road, East Finchley, London, N2 9ED, United Kingdom
Str. Armeneasca 28/1, office 1, Chisinau MD-2012, Republic of Moldova, Europe
Printed at: see last page
ISBN: 978-620-8-30148-4

SUMMARY

Introduction. *Ageing is a universal phenomenon that involves changes in the organism, including the oral cavity of older adults.* ***Objective: To*** *characterise older adults with oral mucosal lesions associated with the use of removable prostheses* ***Methodological design:*** *An observational, descriptive, cross-sectional study was carried out in older adults. Variables: age, sex, oral mucosal lesions, smoking habits, type of prosthesis, material used, time of use, frequency of use, prosthesis hygiene, prosthesis condition. The study population was the older adults who attended the health area, 1392, and the sample selected by non-probabilistic intentional sampling by criteria was 60 older adults.* ***Results:*** *Predominant age was 60 to 69 years, female sex, subprosthetic stomatitis, smoking, total prosthesis, acrylic material, use from 6 to 11 years, frequency of continuous use, poor hygiene and poor prosthetic condition.* ***Conclusions:*** *Older adults between 60 and 69 years of age of female sex predominated. The most frequent lesions were subprosthetic stomatitis and fissured epulis. The main risk factors were smoking, acrylic upper total dentures, time of use from 6 to 11 years, frequency of continuous use, inadequate hygiene and poor condition of the appliance. The highest correlations were found with the type of prosthesis, the material used and the condition of the prosthesis.*

INDEX

INTRODUCTION

Ageing is a universal, dynamic, irreversible, inevitable and progressive phenomenon involving morphological, functional and biochemical changes in the organism. In spite of the gradual alteration manifested, old age is to be considered as a special stage of life.[1 22 22].

The definition of ageing, from a demographic point of view, is related to the increase in the proportion of older people in relation to the rest of the population. The phenomenon is also associated not only with an increase in the proportion of the elderly, but also with a decrease in the proportion of children and young people aged 0-14 years, which has an impact on the economy, the family, services, human capital replacement, social security and on the high costs of medical/epidemiological care.

According to data from the Pan American Health Organisation (PAHO), the world population is ageing by 1.7% annually and it is expected that by 2025 there will be approximately 1100000000 of people over 60 years of age in the world; of this total, according to the Latin American Demographic Centre, 82000000 will be in Latin America.

Latin American and Caribbean ageing has been very rapid and will be even more so. There are countries in different stages of demographic transition; some, such as Bolivia, Guatemala and Haiti, have incipient population ageing; others, such as Uruguay, Argentina, Barbados and Cuba, have advanced ageing.

Cuba is one of the oldest countries in Latin America, with a life expectancy of 78.9 years for men and 80 years for women. By 2050, Cubans are expected to enjoy the oldest average age on the planet, with the economic and social implications that this condition entails.

At the territorial level, there are 8 provinces with demographic dependency ratio values above the national average (613), among which Villa Clara stands out as the province with the highest number of potentially inactive persons per thousand persons aged 15 to 59 (654). In contrast, the territory with the lowest value for this indicator is Artemisa, with 574.[3]

Tooth loss is one of the fundamental characteristics of ageing; the elderly accept it as something inevitable, which is why tooth loss is a health problem in the elderly. It is suggested that tooth loss is not a characteristic of age, but a sign of poor oral health of the patient through a multifactorial process that includes biological, psychological, environmental and patient-related factors due to different causes such as: dental caries, periodontopathies, poor oral hygiene, trauma and poor treatment.

Removable dental prostheses are a treatment alternative to replace missing teeth, but they can also cause damage to the supporting tissues, due to different factors that are considered risk factors such as advancing age, use of the prosthetic appliance for 10 or more years, poor oral and prosthetic hygiene, allergies, immunological problems, poor quality of the prosthetic material, among others [1].

A removable prosthetic appliance is an artificial element whose main function is to restore the anatomy of one or more teeth, as well as to replace functions of the oral cavity such as phonetics and mastication. The rehabilitation of a person using removable dental prostheses is an adaptive process involving a variety of local and systemic tissue changes, on which the success of the prosthetic treatment will depend. Poorly fabricated or poorly maintained prosthetic appliances that have lost their qualities through continued use have contributed to the development of oral lesions. [11]

Oral lesions due to dental prostheses are a problem that affects a large number of older adults worldwide and present several risk factors that affect the oral mucosa. These risk factors generate the appearance of lesions in the oral mucosa, which can be caused by the prolonged use of dental prostheses and their poor preservation, which causes oral lesions to develop easily, but there are patients who do not renew their prostheses and have some type of repair, causing discomfort, pain and instability that can generate intimate contact with the oral mucosa and favour the appearance of these lesions. Likewise, these appearances also can be caused by traumatic circumstances, poor oral hygiene, poor fitting of dentures and reduced salivary flow; taking into account these risk factors, dental professionals should have adequate knowledge about the oral health of older adults who wear dentures because these patients are always undergoing different oral health treatments.[1212].

The presence of lesions of the oral mucosa affects people's general state of health. This is because they are cumulative or progressive pathologies that lead to very complex physiological disorders that can affect the style of eating, the way of communicating, appearance, sometimes causing pain and discomfort. The most frequent area for the development of lesions is the area that maintains constant contact with the internal part of the prosthesis. [13]

Oral lesions have a higher incidence in the older adult population and this is related to the physiological degenerative changes that occur with ageing and to the existence of greater tooth loss, which translates into a greater need to use dental prostheses to maintain masticatory and aesthetic functions. [1]

Oral mucosal lesions are more frequent in elderly people with old or defective dental prostheses and within these, chronic mucosal alterations provide an exceptional entry point for the action of known carcinogens, such as those contained in tobacco, alcohol and other as yet unknown carcinogens. [1]

In order to reduce the prevalence of oral diseases in the elderly, it is necessary to provide them with the necessary knowledge to maintain health and prevent disease, starting with an educational diagnosis to identify learning needs and carry out interventions that can increase knowledge and subsequently achieve a change in attitudes. Oral health is an indispensable condition of the human being, an important source of quality of life; achieving it is only possible with the appropriation and assimilation of knowledge that makes the individual responsible for the care of his or her own. Older adults frequently present poor condition of their dental prostheses and the consequences that this causes in the masticatory system, perhaps due to a lack of knowledge or communication, they are unaware of this and live with it, increasing the problem more and more. The real situation regarding the use of dental prostheses, the lesions in the oral mucosa caused by them and the presence of risk factors that condition the appearance or aggravation of these, are not visibly described and quantified, nor is the relationship between them, even though they are current evidence that does not go unnoticed during the practice of dental care. Due to the increase in oral mucosa lesions caused by removable prostheses in older adults at the Policlínico de Manacas, we propose to carry out this research in order to provide an answer to the following scientific problem:

What characterises Older Adults with lesions in the oral mucosa associated with the use of removable prostheses in the Manacas polyclinic in the municipality of Santo Domingo, Villa Clara province?

OBJECTIVES

General objective:

To characterise older adults with oral mucosal lesions associated with the use of removable prostheses in the Manacas health area from January 2023 to March 2024.

Specific objectives:

1. Distribute the sample according to age and sex

2. To identify injuries associated with the use of removable prostheses in older adults attending dental consultations.
3. To determine risk factors associated with oral mucosal lesions in older adults with dentures.
4. Relate risk factors to lesions affecting the oral mucosa.

THEORETICAL FRAMEWORK

General aspects of ageing:

Ageing is one of the few characteristics that unifies and defines all human beings. It is considered a universal phenomenon, a dynamic, irreversible, inevitable and progressive process, involving a number of physiological changes, mostly simply a decline in the function of the organism as a whole. Of all the evolutionary stages, old age is the one that causes the most limitations in human beings, since it is when different capacities, both intellectual and physical, begin to be lost, and these begin to be accentuated from the age of 60 onwards. 15 Ageing generates a series of changes in the social status, sensory perception, cognitive and motor functions of individuals. At the oral health level, there are also changes in oral tissues and functions, and changes secondary to extrinsic factors, with increased tooth loss due to periodontal disease, caries and oral mucosal lesions.[15]

Changes in the oral cavity of the older adult:

Most of the changes in the oral cavity that occur as a person ages are small and less obvious, making it difficult to distinguish true normal physiological changes from subclinical disease processes.[15]-Lips: The loss of teeth and muscle elasticity causes the orbicularis oris muscle of the lips to become unsupported and consequently have a flaccid appearance (muscular hypotonicity). This causes the skin of the lips to wrinkle inwards. In this way, the chin appears pronounced, known as pseudoprognathism.[16]-Teeth: The older adult undergoes natural wear and tear as a result of chewing without causing discomfort. The most common dental changes associated with age include: occlusal attrition, recession, pulp fibrosis and decreased cellularity. [17,18]-Enamel: The enamel becomes opaque, which causes the dental organs to appear dull, dull and darker in colour. 3With advancing age, enamel tends to become more brittle and susceptible to cracking, fissuring and thus fracture. Darkening and pigmentation have been described that may be caused by absorption of organic material. [17,18] Dentine: There is a change in colour due to the ageing process itself and there is a very noticeable change produced by the replacement of the original dentine by the so-called "repair dentine", which causes the teeth to adopt a yellow tone. These changes cause the teeth to become more fragile due to increased dentine mineralisation.[17]

-Changes caused by tooth loss: The loss of teeth unbalances the distribution of compressive forces along the supporting tissues, causing disorders in the remaining teeth, as the masseter muscle compresses food with a force of 200 kg/cm2. The excess and unbalanced occlusal forces also cause the root cementum to increase in volume in the apical area of the tooth, causing varying degrees of hypercementosis. As the teeth lose their support, the facial musculature is lost, which conditions the typical appearance of the elderly person's face.[15]

-Periodontium: In the gingival aspect, the gingiva is pale pink due to the decrease in blood supply due to the obturation of the submucosal capillaries. Tissue recession occurs, leaving part of the dental root uncovered. In the periodontal tissue there is a decrease in the sensitivity of its fibres that sometimes does not allow pain to be felt, which added to the decrease in manual or psychomotor dexterity, generates the presence and accumulation of dental plaque that leads to serious periodontal problems and cervical dental caries. As a consequence of the problems in the hard and periodontal tissues, serious edentulism is evident, affecting not only masticatory function, but also phonation, self-esteem and aesthetics.**[15]**

-Mucosa: The buccal mucosa becomes thinner, smoother and its appearance is oedematous, with a loss of elasticity and stippling, making it more prone to

lesions, basically due to changes in the epithelium and connective tissue.[15]
-Tongue: With regard to the changes observed in the tongue, there is atrophy of the superficial epithelium, especially on the dorsum, a smooth appearance with loss of filiform papillae, problems with the sense of taste due to a decrease in the number and density of the sensitive nerve endings and a decrease in the taste corpuscles.[16]
-Salivary glands: With ageing there is an atrophy of acinar tissue and a proliferation of ductal products, which is why the major and minor salivary glands go through a process of degenerative changes as the body ages.[16]
-Saliva: During ageing, saliva production is not compromised. It is thought that this is due to the functional reserve capacity of the glands, however, on occasions, its quality and quantity may be affected, associated with the consumption of medicines or treatments with cytotoxic chemotherapy, radiation and other factors.[16]
-Alveolar bone: Ageing is associated with a progressive reduction in bone volume, a manifestation of osteoporosis, which occurs more frequently in edentulous patients with alveolar process and basal bone. This is increased by the lack of dentures, which decreases the vertical dimension and abnormal upward and forward postures of the mandible. Alveolar bone loss is more extensive and occurs more rapidly in the mandible than in the maxilla. [17,18]
-Musculature: Muscle ageing in the stomatognathic system may be related to the depletion of stem cells with age, as well as the occurrence of vascular remodelling, which may be responsible for changes in muscle function. [15]

Edentulism

Among the problems that can be found in this stage of life is edentulism, which is considered a public health problem affecting millions of people around the world, considered a physical disability that affects functions such as eating, speaking and interacting with people. There are many factors that cause this type of problem, especially in older adults. Some of these may be biological, environmental or other types of factors that are related to the patient.

The solution to edentulism is prosthetic rehabilitation, a dental prosthesis (dental plate) is defined as one that aims to adequately replace the crown portions of teeth, replacing them and their associated parts, when they are missing or absent, with artificial means capable of restoring masticatory, aesthetic and phonetic function. The fitting of a prosthesis involves a series of changes and a process of adaptation. Once this period has passed, the patient may have some difficulties when using the prosthesis for different reasons that may be related to problems during mastication, misalignment of the prosthesis, lesions in the oral mucosa, among others.[19]

Lesions of the oral mucosa:

Lesions are alterations that modify the mucosal surface causing changes in colour, texture, swelling and loss of surface integrity. They interfere with everyday functions such as swallowing, communication and chewing. They present symptoms such as burning, pain and irritation, which cause discomfort to patients and interfere with their quality of life. [2]

Classification of oral lesions associated with the use of removable prostheses:

Oral lesions associated with the use of removable prostheses are classified as acute, chronic and progressive. Acute lesions appear as a result of the use of a new, poorly adapted prosthesis, which exerts pressure on the tissues, causing pain and the appearance of ulcerations. Chronic lesions are the result of the instability of prostheses that gradually produce slight friction and these are persistent over time. 20

Subprosthetic stomatitis:

Subprosthetic stomatitis is a chronic inflammatory condition affecting the oral mucosa that is closely related to dental prostheses. It is characterised by oedema, congestion, hyperemia and petechiae. In some patients it is asymptomatic, which leads to a lack of awareness of its existence. [20]

According to González and collaborators it is classified:

- Grade I. Hyperemic spots.

- Grade II. Diffuse erythema.

- Grade III. Granular inflammation or papillary inflammation. This is the most definite lesion.[21] Causes: It is suggested that mechanical factors including traumatic, due to irritation from rubbing of the bases mismatched to the maxilla, poor oral hygiene as well as systemic diseases. [21]

Fibromatous marginal hyperplasia (fissured epulis)

Fissured epulis (FE) traumatic prosthetic fissure tumour or inflammatory fibrous hyperplasia is a hyperplastic growth of mucosa in the gingiva or vestibular sulcus, in contact with the edge of a denture giving it a cleft or figured appearance. [21]

Its occurrence is more common in patients with resorbed alveolar ridges due to the deepening of the prosthesis in the sulcus. Its presence not only causes pain and discomfort but also affects the aesthetic mastication and general condition of the patient. [20]

Types of Fissured Epulis

Fibromatous Epulis: This is a well-defined formation with a homogeneous surface and fibrous appearance; it is poorly vascularised and, when it has evolved for a long time, it may have calcified foci in its central part. They may be isolated or multiple. [22]

-Granulomatous Epulis: It arises from an exaggerated proliferation of granulation tissue, as a mechanism of tissue repair, the organisation of granulation tissue is aborted by the continuous proliferation of endothelial cells stimulated by a foreign body such as a tooth fragment or a bone spicule left in the alveolus after tooth extraction, sometimes caused by amalgam fragments left traumatizing the gingiva after a careless filling.[22] Treatment includes immediate removal of the maladjusted prosthesis. Topical application of palliative medication is recommended, but surgical removal of the lesion cannot be postponed, either by conventional surgery or by laser.

The pain postoperative pain e inflammation usually are minimal. The histopathological analysis is of great importance. [23]

Traumatic ulcers:

Lesion that presents as a solution of continuity of the tissue due to loss of substance. Necrosis of the tissue is observed, greyish-white in colour, with indurated or irregular borders and circumscribed by an erythematous area.[20]

Traumatic ulcers are common on the tongue, buccal mucosa and lower lip, but other areas of the oral region can also be affected depending on their aetiology. These ulcers are the result of iatrogenic injuries committed by the dentist when making dental prostheses. These lesions vary in size and severity, are characterised by a white or yellowish central area and are surrounded by an erythematous halo. Patients report mild to severe pain that lasts approximately 7 to 10 days and affects their ability to perform daily activities and therefore their quality of life is diminished.[20]

If the main cause of these lesions is a poorly adapted prosthesis, the dentist must correct the prosthetic appliance by providing relief in the areas causing the trauma, or replace the dental prosthesis with a new, correctly made one. After correction of the prosthesis the ulcer should heal within 15 days.[20]

Leukoplakia:

Oral keratosis or oral mucosal leukoplakia (OML) is a white patch or plaque that cannot be characterised clinically or histopathologically with another disease.[21] Leukoplakia may appear as a single, localised, diffuse lesion occupying large areas of the buccal mucosa. Its clinical appearance is very heterogeneous; it can vary from macular, smooth, slightly whitish, translucent areas to distinctly white, raised, thick, firm plaques with a rough, fissured surface. They are usually asymptomatic, but some patients may present with a slight burning sensation.[24] This condition can present clinically in multiple forms depending on the clinical pattern, the extent of the lesion and its location within the oral cavity. Two clinical forms are currently considered: homogeneous and non-homogeneous. The distinction between the two is exclusively clinical, based on the colour of the lesion and its morphological characteristics which are related to its evolution. [25] The causes of lesions in the oral cavity are multifactorial, including the combined effects of predisposing and exogenous causal factors, such as tobacco, alcohol, poor oral hygiene, irritation from dentures and others.[25]

Erythroplasia:

An intensely red spot that cannot be defined clinically or pathologically as any other definable disease. 26,27,28,29, 30Clinically, there are two forms of oral erythroplasia: homogeneous and non-homogeneous. The former appears as a red, velvety, smooth lesion with a well-defined border, and the non-homogeneous form shows red areas alternating with white areas of granular or mottled appearance, with irregular surfaces and easy bleeding. 26,27,28,29,30 There are different clinicopathological factors that may influence the appearance of this pathology, such as advanced age and female sex; or environmental aetiological factors, such as tobacco consumption and alcohol intake, chewing tobacco or betel quid; location of lesions and presence of epithelial dysplasia; diets poor in antioxidants (vitamins C, E and beta-carotene); viral infections (human papillomavirus and others); occupational exposure to carcinogens and endogenous causal factors (genetic and hereditary factors). [29,30,31,32, 33]

Risk factors and their relationship to oral lesions

There are several risk factors that lead to the development of oral lesions, and many of them are related to age, the older the person the more likely he or she is to wear dentures. Inadequate lifestyle, poor oral hygiene, use of the prosthesis beyond its useful life, poor patient engagement, predisposing pathologies and factors related to prosthesis making and fitting all play a role in the development and occurrence of oral lesions.[20]

Age

The biological age of an individual is the result of biological maturation processes, and is therefore directly related to this. In addition, the organic and physiological development of the organism is evident, in which genetic and environmental characteristics intervene and determine the individual's state of maturation.[34]

The occurrence of paraprosthetic lesions is related to age, since the more years of life one lives, the greater the possibility of using prostheses, and ageing increases the risk of oral mucosa alterations and disorders, as a consequence of the accumulation of internal physiological factors that cause diseases, which induce biochemical, functional and structural changes. Therefore, the likelihood of developing oral mucosal lesions increases with increasing age.[6,35]

Sex

Sex encompasses biologically determined characteristics, including chromosomal, genetic, anatomical, anatomical, reproductive and physiological traits, thus classifying living beings into male/male and female/female.[36]

Gender is related to oral lesions because females are more affected by the greater number of psychological events associated with hormonal changes that influence them such as: pregnancy, menopause and also their greater concern for aesthetics means that they are more likely to seek rehabilitative treatment.[4]

Smoking

Smoking is a chronic addictive disease, one of the leading causes of morbidity and mortality worldwide, appearing in developed and developing countries. There are a large number of chemical components contained in cigarettes and free radicals, showing that there are no harmless minimum doses for the active smoker or the passive smoker, causing damage at the cellular level.[26,37]

Smoking is a risk factor for the development of malignant and premalignant neoplastic lesions in the oral cavity. The epithelial cells lining the oral mucosa react as defence mechanisms to the stimulus of smoke and combustion, as well as to the chemical-toxic substances that come from them. They manifest themselves as lesions ranging from leukoedema, nicotinic hyperkeratosis, epithelial fibrosis, precancerous lesions, carcinomas in situ, to the development of true malignant neoplasms.[38]

Types of prostheses

-Total prosthesis: will rehabilitate by artificial means all the natural teeth and their associated missing parts. They can be upper and lower or both at the same time, being built with acrylic resins or metal and acrylic resins.[39]

-Partial prosthesis: rehabilitates one or more missing natural teeth and their associated parts, or part of the crown of some teeth but not all of them. [39]

According to the form of retention and placement: The Partial Prosthesis can be:

-Removable Partial Prosthesis.

-Fixed Partial Prosthesis.[39]

The Removable Partial Denture: is constructed in such a way that it can be removed from its position by the wearer or the operator without any damage to the denture or the supporting teeth.[39]

The Fixed Partial Prosthesis: is a restoration that, once it has been made, placed and fixed in position on the supporting teeth that provide its retention, cannot be removed by the wearer or the operator without deterioration of the prosthesis and possible damage to the supporting teeth.[39]

Classification of prostheses according to the material of manufacture:

-Acrylic prostheses: As the name suggests, these are made of acrylic material, a type of rigid plastic that mimics the colour of gum. These prostheses are normally used in patients who have already lost a considerable number of teeth.[40]

-Metallic prosthesis: This is composed of a prosthetic base and a rigid structure made of metal alloys, generally cobalt-chromium (Co-Cr), which favours the three biomechanical pillars of this type of prosthesis: retention, stability and support. It is intended to preserve the remaining biological tissues in the long term.

The prosthetic base is made of acrylic resin (polymethylmethacrylate - PMMA) and is accompanied by artificial teeth that can be made of acrylic or ceramic, restoring aesthetics and phonation to the patient.[40]

Both the metal framework and the prosthetic base material have clinical disadvantages. The metal may exhibit galvanic corrosion when patients have amalgam or gold restorations, due to the interaction of saliva with the metal ions released from the prosthetic material. In addition, CoCrMo metal alloy may cause allergic reactions in the oral mucosa.[40]

Acrylic resin is in direct contact with the oral mucosa of patients; depending on the processing technique, this material may show surface irregularities and favour the adhesion and proliferation of microorganisms, mainly Candida albicans. This pathogen is considered the main cause of prosthetic stomatitis, defined as an inflammatory process of the oral mucosa that supports the prosthesis and appears when the patient has inadequate oral hygiene both on the surface of the prosthesis and on the surrounding mucosa.[40,41]

Time of use of stomatological prostheses:

Patients should be aware that dental prostheses are not made forever, but must be replaced with new ones from time to time, as they wear out and deteriorate, and oral conditions change. Periodic check-ups are important, even in the totally edentulous, for the maintenance of the health of the oral tissues.[10]

The replacement of a dental prosthesis is assessed after approximately 5 years of use, when its functionality and whether there is any damage are determined. The basic criteria that are taken into account to determine the fabrication of a new dental prosthesis are as follows: [10]

-The lack of stability and retention is evident: if there are movements of more than 2 mm in the transverse direction or if the prosthesis does not resist the slightest movement in the vertical direction.

-When a stomatological prosthesis has little extension, which compromises the basic biomechanical principles.

-When food is trapped between the bases and the seating mucosa.

-If there are defects, such as cracks, pits, fractures or loss of teeth, loss of continuity of the prosthetic base, excessive wear of the occlusal surfaces of the teeth.

-Occurrence of injuries related to the dental prosthesis in use. [1]0

The longer the prosthesis is in use, the greater the probability of its misalignment in the mouth becomes more evident, due to the changes that the structures that support it undergo, as well as those that occur in the prosthetic devices themselves, when the prosthesis is worn. gradually deteriorate their usefulness by influencing the development of oral lesions.[10]

Poorly made or inadequately maintained dentures, which have inevitably lost their qualities because the person continues to wear them beyond the required time, contribute to oral tissue damage.[35]

Frequency of use of dental prostheses:

Overnight the denture should be placed in a cleaning solution with water, after brushing, this helps to prevent sub-prosthetic stomatitis and the possible risk of pneumonia events in people who are at a higher risk of developing pneumonia. In this way, the tissues rest for a few hours from the pressure they may be subjected to due to the use of the prosthesis. In addition, removing dentures to sleep at night and leaving them to soak helps prevent denture deformation or cracking.[42]

The continuous use of prostheses prevents the buccal mucosa from receiving the necessary rest from the hystastic changes caused by the rehabilitative apparatus, it also causes degeneration of the salivary glands and mechanical blockage of the excretory ducts, thus reducing salivary secretion, its pH and the buffering action of saliva, which favours the accumulation of dentobacterial plaque. This is why many researchers attach great importance to the time of daily use and recommend a break of six to eight hours a day, so that the tissues can oxygenate, recover and the tongue can achieve self-cleaning.[10]

Hygiene of dental prostheses:

Scientific literature recognises different means to sanitise dentures such as brushing (mechanical method), ultrasound and chemical agents and that the combination of these means is the best option to reduce biofilm and microorganism colonies on the denture surface. Brushing remains the practice of most common hygiene used by prosthesis wearers and that most do not comply with the recommendations on hygiene frequency, time and mode of use of the prosthetic device.[43]

Denture wearers must take extreme care of oral hygiene, it is recommended t o clean the mouth by brushing after each main meal of the day and rinsing with water afterwards. When the rehabilitation is partial, special care must be taken to ensure that the remaining natural teeth, gums, tongue and palate are cared for due to the contact of the denture with them.[44]

Poor hygiene leads to the proliferation of bacteria in the oral cavity and in the prosthetic appliance in partially edentulous patients, can cause caries in the teeth and periodontitis, degenerating the supporting tissues. In fully edentulous patients, it can lead to the accumulation of biofilms on the artificial teeth and on the internal base of the prosthesis, causing lesions and infections in the oral cavity.[45]

Poor condition of dental prostheses:

The physical condition of the prosthetic appliance is an important element in the maintenance of oral health. The poor physical condition of the prosthesis causes various injuries to the rims and buccal mucosa, which worsen as the prosthesis is worn for longer, and is a frequent reason for consultation in dentistry.[43]

When there is a misalignment of the removable prosthesis, irritation can occur that initially causes symptoms such as pain, and the irritation can progress and develop into a pathology that is more difficult to treat.[45]

Procedure and order of oral examination [46]

1- Lip: The exploration of the lip starts from the skin to the mucosa, from one corner to the other and the height to the vestibular sulcus, which is explored together with the vestibular or labial gum up to the canine area. Bimanual palpation will reveal any signs of alterations in the accessory salivary glands, the insertion of the frenulae and the normal consistency of the gum and lip. Mucosa of the cheek: Start on the right side, from the commissure to the retromolar space, which is thoroughly explored; also the rest of the vestibular sulcus and the labial gingiva.

Normal structures such as the termination of the parotid duct, linea alba, ectopic sebaceous glands, occasional dark spots of ethnic origin and the other usual structures in the area should be remembered; the manoeuvre is repeated on the left side.

2- Palate: In this case, the hard palate, the soft palate with the uvula and the anterior pillars as well as the palatal gingiva were included in one examination block. The palatal papilla, the median raphe, the palatal roughness, the mouth of the accessory mucous gland ducts and occasionally the palatal torus should be remembered.

3- Mobile tongue: The dorsal side, edges and apex of the tongue were explored. Check tongue mobility by instructing the patient to project the tongue and move it in all directions.

Bidigital palpation of the dorsal surface and edges was performed, looking for nodules or indurations. For this purpose, the lingual vertex can be grasped with gauze. In this region, filiform, fungiform, fenestrated and foliaceous papillae, medial rhomboid glossitis and lingual fissure and sulcus can usually be identified.

4- Floor of the mouth: With the aid of a depressor or mouth mirror, the floor of the mouth, the ventral aspect of the tongue and the lingual gingiva were examined. For inspection of these sites, instruct the patient to place the apex of the tongue on the hard palate.

For bidigital palpation of the floor of the mouth the index finger of one hand is placed under the chin and the finger of the other hand palpates the anterior floor of the mouth on each side.

The anatomical formations of these sites include: the outlet of the sublingual and submandibular salivary gland ducts, lingual frenulum, prominent sublingual glands, mandibular torus, internal oblique line and apophysis genis (line of insertion of the muscles of the floor of the mouth). Accessory salivary glands may be found on the ventral side of the tongue.

5- Root or base of the tongue and oropharynx: Inspect the root or base of the tongue and the rest of the oropharynx, using the mouth or laryngeal mirror warmed to above body temperature, while pulling the tip of the tongue forwards and downwards with a gauze pad. With the index finger, feel the base of the tongue and the rest of the buccopharynx in a U-shaped movement. The following structures should be identified here: palatine, lingual and pharyngeal tonsils, lymphoid vegetations at the base of the tongue and the vallecula.

METHODOLOGICAL DESIGN

An observational, descriptive, cross-sectional, descriptive study was conducted in adults over 60 during the period January 2023 to March 2024. The study population consisted of all patients over 60 years of age who attended the dentist's office, a total of 1392.For the selection of the sample, a non-probabilistic purposive sampling by criteria was applied, which was taken into consideration: The sample thus consisted of 60 older adults.

Inclusion criteria:

- Older adults with removable total or partial dentures who attend or attend the practice and show their consent to participate in the research (Annex 1).

Exclusion criteria:

- Older adults with health conditions that do not allow them to participate in research

Methods used in the research:

The scientific method was used as a way to carry out the research and to study the essence of the phenomenon.

Theoretical methods:

Analytical - synthetic: It was used for the interpretation of the results of the empirical methods and for the systematisation of the bibliographical study.

Inductive - deductive: Inductive and deductive reasoning made it possible, with the elements related to the information on the injuries present, to arrive at generalities and their determination made it possible to arrive at particularities in the development of the same.

Historical-logical: The historical was used to study the real trajectory of phenomena and events in the course of their history, and the logical investigated the general laws of the functioning and development of the investigated phenomena.

Empirical Methods:

Document analysis: this was used to compile background information on the subject to be studied, taking into account up-to-date documents of recognised scientific rigour

Questionnaire: With the objective of obtain information on socio-demographic variables and variables related to the use of prostheses (Annex 2).

Clinical observation method was used in the clinical examination of each patient in the consultation. To avoid observational bias, data collection and clinical examinations were carried out exclusively by the author under the guidance of the tutor during the time the research lasted. The information obtained was recorded on a data form (Annex 3).

Procedure

Once the necessary regulations had been complied with to begin the investigation, the objectives of the investigation were explained to the patients and informed consent was requested (Appendix 1). Subsequently, a brief questionnaire was administered in the consultation room (Appendix 2) with the aim of obtaining information on socio-demographic variables and variables related to the use of prostheses. Next, an oral examination was carried out in order to identify the presence of oral lesions associated with the use of dental prostheses. The information obtained was entered into an information collection form (Annex 3).

The patients included in the investigation underwent an oral physical examination in a dental chair with the classification set including a mouth mirror, forceps and explorer. It was further carried out the examination of the dental prosthesis by observing it inside and outside the oral cavity

The technical examination of the stomatological prostheses was carried out to determine their condition, taking into account the presence of fractures, wear and misalignment of the prostheses, which was determined by checking their retention and stability in vertical, transversal and sagittal movement. The time and frequency of use of the prosthetic devices was investigated, as well as their hygiene.

Operationalisation of the variables.

Variable	Ranking	Operationalisation		
		Definition	Scale	Indicator
Groups age groups	Discrete quantitative interval-based	According to age at the time of the research	60-69 years 70-79 years 80 and over	Frequency
Sex	Qualitative nominal dichotomous	See will be taken primary sexual characteristics shall be taken into account present	Male Female	Frequency
Oral mucosal lesions	Qualitative Nominal Qualitative Polytomous	According to clinical characteristics of the lesions from on mucosa mucosa	Leukoplakia Erythroplakia Traumatic injuries Cracked epulis	Frequency

		That can be found at collected At oral examination	Subprosthetic stomatitis		
Habit from	Qualitative	According to consumption	Diary: when the		Frequency
smoking	nominal	Usual from	patient smokes all		
	polytomics	any	the days		
		product from	Eventually:		
		tobacco	when the patient		
			smokes 2 or 3 times a year		
			the week		
			Non-smoking: when the		
			patient no		
			Presents the habit		
			smoking		
Type from	Qualitative	According to type from	Total	Top	Frequency
prosthesis	nominal	Prosthesis from		Inferior	
	polytomics	Agreement a its	Partial	Top	
		characteristics		Inferior	
		anatomical			
Material for	Qualitative	According to material	-Metal		Frequency
tailoring	nominal	employed in the	-Acrylic		
From on	polytomics	Tailoring of	-Acrylic	with	
prostheses		apparatus	retainers		
			metallic		
Time of Use of the prosthesis	Quantitative nominal polytomous	Depending on the weather That you carry the prosthesis	:S of 5 years 6 to 11 years 12 and over		Frequency

		installed		
		Referred to to	Continuous : when	Frequency
		Time that	the patient does not	
Frequency of use of the prosthesis	Qualitative nominal dichotomous	the patient remains with the prosthesis. See considered:	removes the prosthesis in the evening hours Discontinuous: when the patient withdraws	
			The prosthesis at	
			night time	
			Inadequate:yes	Frequency
		It was assessed the	there is repository	
		Presence of	hard and/or soft in	
Hygiene of the prosthesis	Qualitative nominal dichotomous	hard deposit and soft at the dental prosthesis dentures,	the maxillary and/or mandibular prosthesis. Adequate: yes no	
		was considered:	there is warehouses	
			hard and soft in	
			its surface	
		During on		Frequency
		Examination clinical examination	Bad: if it presented	
		The following were assessed	fractures, wear and tear	
Status of the prosthesis	Qualitative Nominal polytomics	prostheses taking at the state counts	and/or misaligned Regular :if it was slightly	
		Physical from on	misaligned	
		same .	Good:yesno	
		considered	had no	
			of the conditions previous	

Information processing

Data collection was carried out by the author of the study during the entire research period to avoid information bias.

A database designed for the study was used, summary measures were calculated for qualitative variables (absolute numbers and percentage). Data processing was automated using a Dell PC and specific software. The results for each variable are shown in tables and graphs created for analysis and discussion.

Software used:

- Microsoft Word 2017 word processor.

- Microsoft Excel 2017 Spreadsheet Processor.

- EPIDAT statistical software version 4.2 for Windows

To obtain the distribution of variables according to their attributes and to obtain absolute and relative percentage frequencies, in order to apply descriptive statistics techniques, using the SPSS statistical package, the information will be processed using the Chi-square test, taking as significant values that:

$p < 0.01$ highly significant $p < 0.05$ significant.

$p > 0.05$ no significance. Ethical considerations:

The patients received the necessary information on the characteristics of the study to be carried out. They were asked for their consent in order to obtain their willingness and cooperation in the research, respecting their refusal to participate at all times (Annex 1).

RESULTS

Distribution of patients according to age and sex. Policlínico "Maracas". January 2023 to March 2024.

Age	Male	Sex	Female		Total	
	n%		n%		n%	
60-69 years	12	20,0	23	83,3	35	58,3
70-79 years	7	11,6	10	16,7	17	28,3
80 and over	2	3,4	6	10,0	8	13,4
Total	21	35,0	39	65,0	60	100

Source: Data collection formX^2= 0.613 p = 0.434,

Table 1 shows the distribution of the patients under study according to age group and sex. The female sex was predominant with 39 patients representing 65.0% of the total. The 60-69 age group was the most represented with 35 patients for 58.3% and the 70-79 age group with 17 patients for 28.3% respectively.When applying the chi-square statistical test, no significance was shown as $p>0.05$.

Table 2. Distribution of patients according to age group and presence of oral lesions

Injuries mouth	60-69 years		Age groups 70-79 years80 and over years				Total	
	n%		n	%	n	%	n	%
Leukoplakia	0	0,0	1	1,7	2	3,3	3	5,0
Erythroplasia	2	3,3	1	1,7	0	0,0	3	5,0
Injuries traumatic	3	5,0	1	1,7	0	0,0	4	6,7
Cracked epulis	8	13,4	2	3,3	0	0,0	10	16,7
Stomatitis subprotesis	22	36,7	12	20,0	6	10,0	40	66,7
Total	35	58,3	17	28,3	8	13,4	60	100

Source: Clinical examination and data collection form. X^2= 4.440 p = 0.107

According to the data in table 2, the most frequent oral lesions in patients with removable prostheses were subprosthetic stomatitis with 40 patients (66.7%), fissured epulis with 10 patients (16.7%) and traumatic lesions with 4 patients (6.7%). In terms of age group, the 60-69 years age group was more affected by subprosthetic stomatitis with 22 patients for 36.7%. When applying the chi-square statistical test, significance was not demonstrated a s p>0.05.

Table 3. Distribution of patients according to oral lesions and smoking status

Injuries mouth	Diary		Smoking Eventual		Non-smoking		Total	
	n	%	n	%	n	%	n	%
Leukoplakia	3	5,0	0	0,0	0	0,0	3	5,0
Erythroplasia	1	1,7	0	0,0	2	3,3	3	5,0
Injuries traumatic	1	1,7	0	0,0	3	5,0	4	6,7
Cracked epulis	2	3,3	4	6,7	4	6,7	10	16,7
Stomatitis subprotesis	14	23,3	11	18,3	15	25,0	40	66,7
Total	21	35,0	15	25,0	24	40,0	60	100

Source: Clinical examination and data collection sheet X^2=25.724 p = 0.502

Table 3 describes smoking habits and the presence of oral lesions. A total of 21 patients with oral lesions studied smoke daily (35.0%), while 15 patients (25.0%) smoke occasionally, which is related to the appearance of lesions. All the patients who smoke daily have some kind of oral lesion, predominantly subprosthetic stomatitis with 14 patients (23.3%), 3 patients with leukoplakia (5.0%), 2 patients with fissured epulis (3.3%), 1 patient with erythroplakia (1.7%) and 1 with traumatic lesions (1.7% of the sample). When applying the chi-square statistical test, significance was not demonstrated as p>0.05.

Table 4. Distribution of patients according to oral lesions and type of removable dentures

Injuries mouth	Type of removable dental prosthesis Total prosthesisPartial prosthesis Upper Lower Upper Lower								Total	
	n%		n%		n%		n%		n%	
Leukoplakia	1	1,7	2	3,3	0	0,0	0	0,0	3	5,0
Erythroplasia	1	1,7	0	0	1	1,7	1	1,7	3	5,0
Injuries traumatic	1	1,7	1	1,7	2	3,3	0	0,0	4	6,7
Epulis cracked	3	5,0	2	3,3	2	3,3	3	5,0	10	16,7
Stomatitis subprotesis	21	35,0	2	3,3	13	21,7	4	6,7	40	66,7
Total	27	45,0	7	11,6	18	30,0	8	13,6	60	100

Source: Clinical examination and data collection form. X^2= 4.440p = 0.107

In table 4, total upper dentures predominated in 27 patients for 45.0% followed by partial upper dentures in 18 patients for 30.0%, in both there is a predominance of subprothesis stomatitis lesion with 35.0% and 21.7% respectively. When applying the chi-square statistical test, there is no significance because p>0.05.

Table 5. Distribution of patients according to oral lesions and material used to make the removable dental prosthesis.

Injuries	Clothing material							
mouth	Acrylic		Acrylic with metal retainers		Metal		Total	
	n	%	N	%	N	%	n	%
Leukoplakia	3	5,0	0	0,0	0	0,0	3	5,0
Erythroplasia	3	5,0	0	0,0	0	0,0	3	5,0
Injuries	2	3,3	2	3,3	0	0,0	4	6,7
traumatic								
Epulis	9	15,0	1	1,7	0	0,0	10	16,
cracked								7
Stomatitis	31	51,7	7	11,7	2	3,3	40	66,
subprotesis								7
Total	48	80,0	10	16,7	2	3,3	60	100

Source: Clinical examination and data collection form. X^2= 24.841: 0.119

Taking into account the material used to make the removable dental prosthesis shown in table 5, a predominance of acrylic material was observed in 48 appliances for 80.0%. In this material, subprosthetic stomatitis type lesions predominated with 31 patients for 51.7% and the lesion of fissured epulis with 9 patients for 15.0% of the sample studied. In the case of the acrylic material with metal retainers, 10 patients were found, representing 16.7%, and subprosthetic stomatitis was also the most frequent lesion with 7 patients for 11.7%, and the application of the chi-squared statistical test did not demonstrate significance, since $p>0.05$

Distribution of patients according to oral lesions and time of use of the removable dental prosthesis.

Injuries mouth	Time of use of the removable dental prosthesis 5 and under6 to 11 years12 years and over years						Total	
	n%		n%		N%		n%	
Leukoplakia	0	0,0	2	2,3	1	1,7	3	5,0
Erythroplasia	0	0,0	0	0,0	3	5,0	3	5,0
Injuries traumatic	4	6,7	0	0,0	0	0,0	4	6,7
Cracked epulis	0	0,0	10	16,7	0	0,0	10	16,7
Stomatitis subprotesis	2	3,3	26	43,3	12	20,0	40	66,7
Total	6	10,0	38	63,3	16	26,7	60	100

Source: Clinical examination.X^2=25.52 p : 0.526

Table 6 shows the results of the distribution of patients according to oral lesions and time of use of the removable dental prosthesis. According to the length of time the prostheses had been worn, those between 6 to 11 years prevailed with 38 patients for 63.3%, followed by 12 and more years with 16 patients for 26.7% and finally 5 and less years with 6 patients for 10.0%. In the 6 to 11 years age group, subprosthetic stomatitis type lesions predominated with 26 patients (43.3%) and fissured epulis with 10 patients (16.7%); however, in the 5 and under age group, traumatic lesions predominated with 4 patients (6.7%). When applying the chi-square statistical test, there is no significance as $p>0.05$.

Table 7. Distribution of patients according to oral lesions and frequency of use of the removable dental prosthesis

Oral lesions	Frequency of use of the prosthesis				Total	
	Discontinuous		Continuous			
	n	%	n	%	n	%
Leukoplakia	1	1,7	2	3,3	3	5,0
Erythroplasia	0	0,0	3	5,0	3	5,0
Injuries traumatic	1	1,7	3	5,0	4	6,7
Cracked epulis	4	6,7	6	10,0	10	16,7
Stomatitis subprotesis	9	15,0	31	51,7	40	66,7
Total	15	25,0	45	75,0	60	100

Source: Clinical examination and data collection form. X^2=21.54 p : 0.336

When analysing the frequency of use of the prosthesis as shown in table 7, it was found that 75.0% (45 patients) had continuous use of the prosthesis, while only 25.0% had it removed at some point. When applying the chi-square statistical test, no significance was found, as p>0.05.

Table 8. Distribution of patients according to oral lesions and removable dental prosthesis hygiene

Oral lesions	Hygiene of the prosthesisTotal					
	Adequate		Inadequate			
	n%		n%		n%	
Leukoplakia	2	3,3	1	1,7	3	5,0
Erythroplasia	1	1,7	2	3,3	3	5,0
Injuries traumatic	2	3,3	2	3,3	4	6,7
Cracked epulis	4	6,7	6	10,0	10	16,7
Stomatitis subprotesis	11	18,3	29	48,3	40	66,7
Total	20	33,3	40	66,7	60	100

Source: Clinical examination and data collection form. X^2=21.76 p: 0.344 .

When assessing the hygiene of the prostheses in table 8, it was found that 66.7%, represented by a total of 40 patients, had inadequate hygiene. When applying the chi-square statistical test, no significance was found, as p>0.05.

Table 9. Distribution of patients according to oral lesions and state of removable dental prosthesis

Injuries oral	Condition of removable dental prosthesisTotal GoodFairPoor							
	n	%	n	%	n	%	n	%
Leukoplakia	1	1,7	1	1,7	1	1,7	3	5,0
Erythroplasia	2	3,3	1	1,7			3	5,0
Injuries traumatic	1	1,7	2	3,3	1	1,7	4	6,7
Cracked epulis	3	5,0	5	8,3	2	3,3	10	16,7
Stomatitis subprotesis	9	15,0	5	8,3	27	45,0	40	66,7
Total	16	26,7	14	23,3	31	51,7	60	100

Source: Clinical examination and data collection form. $X^2=20.83$ p : 0.331

In relation to the condition of the prosthesis, table 9 shows that it was poor in 31 patients (51.7%) and fair in 14 (23.3%), of which 27 patients (45.0%) had subprosthetic stomatitis. When applying the chi-square statistical test, significance was not demonstrated as $p>0.05$.

Table 10. Relationship between risk factors and oral mucosal lesions taking into account the chi-square test values achieved.

Risk factors	Oral lesions	
	X^2	P
Smoking	25,724	0,502
Type of prosthesis	4,440	0,107
Material for making up the prosthesis	24,841	0,119
Time of use of the prosthesis	25,52	0,526
Frequency of use of the prosthesis	21.54	0.336
Hygiene of the prosthesis	21.76	0.344
Condition of the prosthesis	20.83	0.331

When relating the studied risk factors and oral mucosa lesions in table 10, taking into account the P values, we observe that the most significant risk factor was the type of prosthesis, followed by the material used to make the prosthesis, the condition of the prosthesis and the frequency of use of the prosthesis, since the P values are closer to 0.00.

DISCUSSION

The growing increase in life expectancy has made the ageing of society a matter of utmost interest due to an increase in diseases related to this process. It is therefore necessary to take into account the individual characteristics and oral health needs of the elderly in order to promote actions to achieve better quality care and satisfaction of this population.[47] In studies carried out by Yero Mier and collaborators[48] in Sancti Spíritus, it was found that the female sex was the most affected with 66%. In addition, the predominant age group was between 60 and 69 years of age, which coincides with the results of the present study. Similar to our research, Rodríguez Baquero[49] and Martínez Gonzáles[50] also found that the female sex was the most representative with 87% and 50% respectively. However, Rodríguez Pimienta[51] found that more men were affected by oral mucosal lesions, with 59.6%. These results may be associated with the fact that women are affected by a greater number of psychological events and hormonal changes that influence them, such as pregnancy and menopause; they are also more concerned about aesthetics, which leads them to seek rehabilitation treatment more frequently. With regard to age, Piña Odio[35] found that patients aged 60 years and over were the most affected, which is in line with our results, as were other researchers[52,53] who found the 60-69 age range to be the most predominant. The study by Ramírez Barrios[5] differs from the results obtained in our study. He found that the age range with the highest number of older adults with oral mucosal lesions was 80 to 85 years with 38.8%. The author considers that oral mucosal lesions caused by dentures are somewhat related to age, as the more years of life, the greater the possibility of need prosthetic rehabilitation. In addition, the physiological changes brought about by ageing deteriorate the organism and its structures, which increases the risk of presenting alterations and affections of the oral mucosa.In the present investigation it was found that the most frequent lesions in the studied population were subprosthetic stomatitis followed by fissured epulis and traumatic ulcer. In terms of age group, the 60-69 age group was found to be most affected by subprosthetic stomatitis. Similar to our result, García Rodríguez[54] observed that subprosthetic stomatitis was present in more than half of those examined with 52.8%. Gonzáles Beriau[1] also showed that the most frequent lesion was subprosthetic stomatitis with 90.2%, where it was more evident in the 65-69 age range with 45.7%. This lesion was followed by fissured stomatitis with 7.8%, coinciding with the present study. In addition, Cruz Sixto and collaborators[52] obtained a high percentage of older adults with subprosthetic stomatitis with 83.2 %, followed by traumatic ulcer with 8.7 %. The results found in the present investigation differ from those of Salazar Gamez[55] who found that the highest prevalence of mucosal lesions caused by dental prostheses was angular cheilitis with 52.5 %, followed by oral candidiasis with 11.9 %.The researcher considers that, despite finding differences in the reviewed studies, in most of them the most frequent lesion was subprosthetic stomatitis, which validates the scientific findings of the study, demonstrating once again that subprosthetic stomatitis is the most prevalent disease of the oral mucosa related to the use of dental prostheses.When analysing our sample, we found that 60 % of patients with oral lesions smoke daily or occasionally, so smoking is somewhat related to the occurrence of oral lesions. Similar to our results, Rodríguez Pimienta and collaborators[51] state that smoking was one of the predominant risk factors with 40.4%

Espasandín González and collaborators[13] stated that oral lesions were more numerous among smokers with 53.75%, figures that differ with great statistical significance from the rest of the harmful habits they studied, with low percentages. These contributions show similarities with those found in our research. No reports were found that differed from our research. The author considers that smoking is one of the most difficult habits for the health professional to control due to the dependence it exerts on the patient. Aspects such as anxiety, the influence of the social environment in which the individual develops, constantly threaten the eradication of this harmful habit. As health professionals, we must insist in every consultation on the importance of eliminating this habit, explaining to patients all the alterations it causes in oral tissues and the predisposition it produces to the appearance of other oral and systemic diseases. We can also provide professional help to patients who come to our services worried about their addiction and refer them to other specialists such as psychologists who can help them eliminate the habit.

A study from 2020 in Pinar del Río[52] states that there was a predominance of patients with total prostheses who presented oral lesions. Ramírez Barrios[5] also states that the greatest affectation was caused by total prostheses for 57.2 %, results that agree with our study. In a study carried out by Eugen[53] it was found that the most common type of prosthesis used by the subjects included was the maxillary partial prosthesis (35.55%), which differs from our study where the most frequent type of prosthesis was the total prosthesis.From the author's point of view, full dentures, especially upper dentures, have a greater number of contact points with the buccal mucosa than full dentures. partial dentures. This is due to the fact that full dentures have a larger seating surface both in the maxilla and in the mandible, so there is a greater probability of causing injuries, which increases in the presence of other risk factors such as continuous use, poor hygiene and poor physical condition of the prosthesis.

According to results published in Colombia by Rodríguez Baquero[49] , oral lesions occurred to a greater extent in acrylic prostheses with 71.4%. Ramírez Barrios[5] stated that the highest percentage of involvement corresponds to acrylic bases in total and partial removable prostheses. These results coincide with those obtained in our research, where prostheses made of acrylic were the most relevant, and no results were found that differed from ours. In the author's opinion, despite the advances that exist in the field of prosthetic rehabilitation with flexible and more aesthetic materials for the manufacture o f dental prostheses, there is no access to these materials in Cuba, which is why acrylics and to a lesser extent metals continue to be used. After some time of use, these materials undergo modifications that can damage the supporting tissues and lead to the appearance of oral lesions. It is therefore necessary to instruct the patient in the proper use and care of the rehabilitating apparatus and its timely replacement to avoid the appearance of this type of pathology.

According to the time of use of the prostheses, prostheses with 6 to 11 years of use prevailed. Similar results were shown by other authors such as Salazar Gamez[55] with a time of use of 6 to 11 years in 50% of the patients, González Beriau[1] with a range of 5 to 9 years of use which is within the limits obtained in our research. In addition, García Rodríguez[54] also obtained a similar result with a time of use of more than 5 years with 40.1%.Other researchers[49,53] showed results that differed from ours with a shorter time of use of the prosthetic device than that observed in our study. From the results obtained, the author considers that despite finding results that differ from the present research, the more years of use a dental prosthesis has been in use, the more likely it is to be deteriorated with wear and tear. fractures, repairs and misalignments, which increase the risk of injury to the oral mucosa.In the research context, most of the patients with oral lesions were wearing their dentures incorrectly, as they were wearing them continuously. A study carried out in Mayabeque[13] in 2021 showed that 48.75 Of the patients with oral lesions, % of them wore the denture continuously and Macias Yen Chong[43] states that most of the patients (78 %) wore the denture all day long (24 hours) and about half of them have clinical signs of subprosthetic stomatitis (46 %), results that coincide with ours.

Garcia Rodriguez[54] also observed that wearing time of more than 5 years and continuous use of prostheses were the most relevant risk factors in his research, which was similar in our study.Based on the results obtained in the previous research, the author believes that it is very important to guide patients about the advantages of allowing the mucosa covered by the prosthesis to rest during sleep time, in order to allow the tissues to oxygenate and recover, as well as giving the tongue and lips the opportunity to perform their self-cleaning action.

In relation to denture hygiene, it was found that the majority of patients with oral lesions did not have adequate hygiene.

Similar to our study, Cruz Sixto[52] shows that 69.3 % of patients had regular or poor prosthesis hygiene. Espasandín González[13] when analysing inadequate and harmful prosthetic habits to the mucosa in the study population, observed a higher number of patients diagnosed with oral lesions among those patients who use prostheses continuously and who have a The results were similar to those of our study, with 48.75 % and 41.25 % of the patients reporting poor oral hygiene and poor prosthesis hygiene, respectively. Yero Mier[48] observed in his research that 65 % of the prostheses showed accumulation of bacterial plaque and food debris, which translates into poor hygiene of the prosthetic appliance, coinciding with our results. No results were found that differed from ours.

The author considers that oral and prosthetic hygiene is one of the factors that could determine oral health, since the accumulation of alba matter and dental plaque, plus the presence of opportunistic microorganisms added to a diminished immune system in the elderly is a determining factor in the development of pathologies in the oral cavity. Furthermore, this high frequency of lesions in the oral mucosa related to the infrequency of hygiene could be related to the insufficient health education activities, in which the patient should be taught the correct way to clean the prosthesis and remaining teeth (if they have them), so that promotion and prevention continue to be the fundamental weapons to avoid diseases. As for the condition of the prosthesis, a large number of patients were in poor condition. Research by Martínez Gonzáles[50] showed that 35% of patients had a poor condition of the prosthesis due to misalignment and excessive mobility. Rodríguez Pimienta[51] and González Frías[56] showed similar results where a large number of patients had maladjusted prostheses with 38.2% and 66% respectively.No study showed differences with the results obtained, which ratifies this risk factor as one of the most related to the appearance of oral lesions. In the opinion of the author of this research, the continuous use of prostheses in a poor state of conservation causes a greater risk of suffering some type of lesion, which coincides with that described by other authors, who point out that when they are misadjusted and in poor condition, it constitutes a risk factor for the development of oral lesions. For this reason, annual control and adjustment should be recommended, as well as nocturnal removal of the dentures, which will help to reduce these lesions. When relating the risk factors and oral mucosal lesions by analysing the P values, we observed that the most frequent risk factor was the type of prosthesis, followed by the material used to make the prosthesis, results similar to those obtained by Piña Odio[3]5 , where total mucosa-supported prostheses were the most significant risk factor. Arias Fernández57 found that smoking was the most significant risk factor, which differs from our study.

CONCLUSIONS

Oral mucosal lesions associated with the use of removable dentures were more frequent in females in the 60-69 age group.

-The pathology with the highest incidence was subprosthetic stomatitis followed by fissured stomatitis and traumatic ulcer.

-The main risk factors were smoking, total upper dentures, acrylic material, wearing time of 6 to 11 years, frequency of continuous wear, inadequate hygiene and poor condition of the appliance.

The most significant relationships were with prosthesis type, prosthesis material and prosthesis condition as they showed P-values closest to 0.00.

BIBLIOGRAPHICAL REFERENCES

1- González-Beriau Y, Marrero-Santana L. Mucosal lesions associated with the use of dental prostheses in older adult patients. Medisur [journal on the Internet]. 2022 [cited 2022 Sep 30]; 20(5):[approx. -864 p.].Available from: http://www.medisur.sld.cu/index.php/medisur/article/view/5480

2- Marín W, Veiga L, Reyes Y, Mesa D. Oral lesions in older adults and risk factors, Policlínico "Dr. Tomás Romay", Havana, Cuba. Rev Haban Cienc Méd [journal on the Internet]. 2017[cited 3 Sep 2022] ; 16 (5): [approx. 13p].Available from: http://www.revhabanera.sld.cu/index.php/rhab/article/view/2070/1897.

3-El Envejecimiento de la Población. Cuba y sus territorios-2022. informed 13 July 2023 [cited 2024 Feb 12] Available from: https://www.infomed.scu.sld.cu/el- envejecimiento-de-la-poblacion-cuba-y-sus-territorios-2022/

4- Vázquez de León Ana Gloria, Palenque Guillemí Ana Isabel, Morales Montes de Oca Teresita de Jesús, Bermúdez Morales Daily Caridad, Barrio Pedraza Teresita de Jesús. Oral mucosal lesions associated with the use of dental prostheses. Medisur [Internet]. 2019 Apr. Available at: http://scielo.sld.cu/scielo.php?script=sci_arttext&pid=S1727-897X2019000200201201&lng=en

5- Ramírez Barrios A, González Méndez FR. Oral disorders and risk factors in older adults with dental prostheses. Rev Ciencias Médicas [Internet]. 2022 [cited: date of access]; 26(4): e5412. Available from: http://revcmpinar.sld.cu/index.php/publicaciones/article/view/5412

6- Morales Pérez YJ, Meras Jáuregui TM, Batista Aldereguia MY. Paraprosthetic soft tissue lesions in patients with total prosthesis. Medicentro Electrónica [Internet]. 2019 Mar [cited 06/01/2022]; 23(1): 19-25. Available from: http://scielo.sld.cu/scielo.php?script=sci_arttext&pid=S1029-30432019000100004&lng=en.

7- Sixto Iglesias MS, Arencibia García E, Labrador Falero DM. Measurement of the level of satisfaction of the clinical services of stomatological prosthesis. Rev Medical Sciences [Internet]. 2018 Apr [cited 06/01/2022]; 22(2): 85-93. Available from: http://scielo.sld.cu/scielo.php?script=sci_arttext&pid=S1561-31942018000200011&lng=en.

8- Torres Lagares D, Gutiérrez Corrales A, Gutiérrez Pérez JL, Serrera Figallo MA. Clinic, aetiopathogenesis and clinical management of pain in osteonecrosis of the jaws. Faculty of Dentistry - University of Seville. Communications to Congresses/Medicine and Health Sciences. 2019 [cited 06/01/2022]; [approx. 16 p.]. Available from: https://www.scientificmedicaldata.com/article.php?o7hkX7RRVmXFKovo06eRK5Hc W/8cyAu+tUYZmzyMfs4.

9- Huamani Cantoral JE, Huamani Echaccaya JL, Alvarado Menacho S. Oral rehabilitation in patients with alteration of the occlusal vertical dimension applying a multidisciplinary approach. Rev Estomatol Herediana [Internet]. 2018 [cited 06/01/2022]; 28(1): 44-55. Available from: http://www.scielo.org.pe/pdf/reh/v28n1/a06v28n1.pdf

10- Lazo Nodarse R, Sariol Pérez D, Hernández Reyes B, Puig Capote E, Rodríguez Rodríguez M, Sanford Ricard M. Stomatological prosthesis as a risk factor for premalignant and malignant lesions in the oral cavity. AMC [Internet]. 2019 Aug [cited 06/01/2022]; 23(4): 487-99. Available from: http://scielo.sld.cu/pdf/amc/v23n4/1025- 0255-amc-23-04-487.pdf.

11- González Feria R k.Characterization of oral lesions in removable prosthesis wearers. Julio Antonio Mella University Teaching Polyclinic. Holguín. 2022. [Thesis] approx 57 Available at: https://tesis.hlg.sld.cu/index.php?P=DownloadFile&Id=2759

12- Pinzón. L, Gaviari, N, Florián. K, Gutiérrez. A. Manifestaciones Orales En Pacientes De La Tercera edad con uso de prótesis dentales [degree thesis]. Bogotá: Antonio Nariño University; 2022. 15p. Available in: http://repositorio.uan.edu.co/bitstream/123456789/7919/1/2023.TG.Pinz%C3%B3nPast or%2CLeydiJhoana.pdf

13- Espasandín González S, González Díaz Y, Reyes Suárez VO, González Casañas BY. Prosthetic aggressions to the oral mucosa in geriatric patients rehabilitated with removable stomatological prostheses. AD [Internet]. Oct 5, 2021 [cited Mar 12, 2024];4(4):79-6. Available from: https://cienciadigital.org/revistacienciadigital2/index.php/AnatomiaDigital/article/view/1 900

14- Vázquez González Juan Alejandro, Ramos González Rosa María, Rodríguez Suárez Sabrina, Fernández Campo Ramona. Oral health knowledge in the elderly. Clinic 10. Polyclinic "Dr. Tomas Romay. Rev.Med.Electron. [Internet]. 2020 Oct [cited 2024 Mar 14]; 42(5): 2248-2261. Available from: http://scielo.sld.cu/scielo.php?script=sci_arttext&pid=S1684-18242020000502248&lng=en

15- Torrecilla-Venegas R, Castro-Gutiérrez I. Effects of ageing on the oral cavity. April 16 [Internet]. 2020 [date of citation]; 59 (278): e819. Available from: http://www.rev16deabril.sld.cu/index.php/16_4/article/view/819

16- Álvarez Muguercia Reyna Zara, González Grasso Aylen, Mustelier Mojena Silvina. Health care to the elderly patient, from the perspective of the disability - aging relationship. Rev Hum Med [Internet]. 2023 Apr [cited 2024 Mar 12] ; 23(1): e2425. Available from: http://scielo.sld.cu/scielo.php?script=sci_arttext&pid=S1727-81202023000100016&lng=en.

17- Tapia Diaz LO, García Delgado F. Dental management of the older adult patient. Lima Peru: Universidad Inca Garcilaso de la Vega; 2021 [cited 23 Sep

2022].Available
from:http://repositorio.uigv.edu.pe/bitstream/handle/20.500.11818/5574/TRACADEMICO_TAPIA%20DIAZ.pdf?sequence=1&isAllowed=y

18- Castellanos J., Diaz L., Lee E. Medicina en odontologia. 3ª. Mexico: El manual moderno; 2015.

19- Tonato-Hidalgo Jeanine Dailyn, Loor-Tobar Nayla Shenoa, Gavilanez-Villamarín Silvia Marisol, Armijos-Moreta Jaime Fernando. Influence of the use of dental prostheses on the quality of life of older adults. Rev. inf. cient. [Internet]. 2022 Dec [cited 2024 Mar 22]; 101(6): e4054. Available from: http://scielo.sld.cu/scielo.php?script=sci_arttext&pid=S1028-99332022000600005&lng=en.

20- Fernández Hernández CP. Oral lesions associated with the use of removable prostheses in older adults. 2023 [cited 29 October 2023].Available from: http://repositorio.ug.edu.ec/handle/redug/66607

21- Santana Garay JC, Atlas de anatomía del complejo buccal. 2nd Edition Editorial de Ciencias Médica, La Habana 2010 p 251-252, 288-293

22- Jaramillo Jiménez TN. Planning and surgical treatment of pre-prosthetic surgeries of the maxillofacial territory. Thesis [Internet]. 2013 [cited 2013 Oct 30, 2023]. Available from: http://repositorio.ug.edu.ec/handle/redug/3639

23- Quesada-Iraizoz L, Denis-Navarro Y, de-Quesada-Suárez L. Fissured epulis of unusually prolonged evolution. Archives of the "General Calixto García" University Hospital [Internet]. 2019 [cited 29 Oct 2023]; 7 (1) :[approx. 4 p.]. Available from: https://revcalixto.sld.cu/index.php/ahcg/article/view/304

24- González González G, Ardanza Zuleta P, Santos Solana L, Denis Alfonso A, Carriera Piloto V, Jourbert-Martir R. et al Rehabilitación protésica estomatológica [Internet]. Editorial ciencias médicas la habana; 2008. p 268-271 .Available at: https://catalogo.hlg.sld.cu/index.php?P=FullRecord&ID=9597

25- Castelnaux MM, Montoya SI, Serguera BY, et al. Clinical and epidemiological characterization of patients with oral leukoplakia. MediSan. 2020;24(01):4-15.available at https://www.medigraphic.com/cgi-bin/new/summary.cgi?IDARTICLE=96037

26- Estrada Pereira Gladys Aída, Agüero Despaigne Liliet Antonia. Clinical and histopathological manifestations of oral erythroplasia in patients who smoke tobacco. Medisur [Internet]. 2023 Aug [cited 2024 Mar 18] ; 21(4): 842-850. Available from: http://scielo.sld.cu/scielo.php?script=sci_arttext&pid=S1727-897X2023000400842&lng=en

27- Eccles K, Carey B, Cook R, Escudier M, Diniz M, Limeres J, et al. Potentially malignant oral disorders: recommendations for primary care management. J Oral Med Oral Surg[Internet]. 2022 [cited 10/4/2023];(38):[approx. 20p]. Available from: https://opmdcare.com/wp-content/uploads/trastornos-orales- potentially-malignant-oral-disorders-recommendations-on-approach-in-primary-care.pdf.

28- Warnakulasuriya S, Kujan O, Aguirre JM, Bagan JV, González MÁ, Kerr AR, et al. Oral potentially malignant disorders: A consensus report from an international seminar on nomenclature and classification, convened by the WHO Collaborating Centre for Oral Cancer. Oral Dis. 2021;27(8):1862-80.

29- Lorenzo AI, Lafuente I, Pérez M, Pérez A, Chamorro CM, Blanco A, et al. Critical update, systematic review, and meta-analysis of oral erythroplakia as an oral potentially malignant disorder. J Oral Pathol Med. 2022;51(7):585-93.

30- Kumari P, Debta P, Dixit A. Oral Potentially Malignant Disorders: Etiology, Pathogenesis, and Transformation Into Oral Cancer. Front Pharmacol. 2022;13:825266 31-Iparraguirre MF, Fajardo X, Carneiro E, Couto PH. Potentially malignant oral disorders. What the dentist should know. Rev Estomatol Herediana [Internet]. 2020 [cited 10/4/2023];30(3):[approx. 11p]. Available from:

http://www.scielo.org.pe/scielo.php?script=sci_arttext&pid=S1019-43552020000300216

32- Tovío EG, Carmona MC, Díaz AJ, Harris J, Lanfranchi HE. Clinical expressions of potentially malignant oral cavity disorders. Integrative review of the literature. Univ Odontol[Internet]. 2018[cited 10/4/2023];37(78):[approx. 32p].

Disponible en: https://revistas.javeriana.edu.co/files-articulos/UO/UO%2037-78%20(2018-I)/231260072005/231260072005_visor_jats.pdf

33- Páramo JT, Rivera DI. Epithelial dysplasias, a diagnostic challenge for the oral pathologist. Rev Odont Mex [Internet]. 2021 [cited 10/4/2023];25(3):[approx. 2p]. Available from: https://www.medigraphic.com/pdfs/odon/uo-2021/uo213a.pdf

34- Gil Suárez Ángel Lázaro, Zaldívar Pérez Bergelino. Study of the biological age in male athletes of the school category. Rev Podium [Internet]. 2021 Aug [cited 2024 Mar 21] ; 16(2): 490-508. Available from: http://scielo.sld.cu/scielo.php?script=sci_arttext&pid=S1996-24522021000200490&lng=en

35- Piña Odio Ibis, Matos Frómeta Katiusca, Barrera Garcell Mayra, Gonzalez Longoria Ramírez Yissel Maurín, Arencibia Flandes María del Pilar. Risk factors related to the paraprosthetic lesions in patients with removable prosthesis. MEDISAN [Internet].

2021 Feb [cited 2024 Mar 19] ; 25(1): 41-50. Available from: http://scielo.sld.cu/scielo.php?script=sci_arttext&pid=S1029-30192021000100041&lng=en.

36- Abad-Colil Felipe, Ramírez-Vélez Robinson, Fernandes-Da Silva Sandro, Ramirez- Campillo Rodrigo. Importance of sex/gender and its distinction in biomedical research. Towards promoc. Health [Internet]. 2019 July [cited 2024 Mar 21] ; 24(2):

11-13. Available from: http://www.scielo.org.co/scielo.php?script=sci_arttext&pid=S0121-75772019000200011&lng=en. https://doi.org/10.17151/hpsal.2019.24.2.2.

37- Renda L, Cruz Y, Parejo D, Cuenca K. Level of knowledge about smoking and its relationship with the oral cavity. Rev Cub Med Mil[Internet]. 2020 [cited 10/4/2023];49(1):[approx. 14p]. Available from: https://revmedmilitar.sld.cu/index.php/mil/article/view/280/443

38- Guerrero Brito Marisleydi, Pérez Cabrera Duniesky, Hernández Abreu Noelí Marta. Premalignant oral lesions in patients with smoking habit. Medicentro Electrónica

[Internet]. 2020 Mar [cited 2024 Mar 23] ; 24(1): 159-164. Available from: http://scielo.sld.cu/scielo.php?script=sci_arttext&pid=S1029-30432020000100159&lng=en.

39- González Hernández Giselle María, Ramos Padrón Adria, Licea Rodríguez Yamilín.Diferentes prótesis y sus usos estomatológicos.2021 [cited 2024 January 11] approx 19p Available from https://aulavirtual.sld.cu/mod/resource/view.php?id=91948 40-Castillo-Pedraza Midian Clara, Inagati Cristiane Mayumi, Wilches-Visbal Jorge Homero. Use of removable partial dentures with thermoplastic acrylic resin: a literature review. Salud, Barranquilla [Internet]. 2023 Apr [cited 2024 Mar 21] ; 39(1): 265-283. Available from: http://www.scielo.org.co/scielo.php?script=sci_arttext&pid=S0120-55522023000100265&lng=en. Epub Nov 18, 2023. https://doi.org/10.14482/sun.39.01.222.315.

41- Mohammed G, Fouda S. Current perspectives and the future of Candida albicans- associated denture stomatitis treatment. Dent Med Probl. 2020;57(1):95-102. Available at: http://www.dmp.umed.wroc.pl/pdf/2020/57/1/95.pdf.

42- Denture Care Guide,12 November 2021,Dental Gazette, [approx 6p] Available at: https://gacetadental.com/2021/11/guia-para-el-cuidado-de- las-protesis-dentales-28333/

43- Macías-Yen Chong Yohana Geomar, Díaz-Pérez Carlos Alberto, Martínez-Rodríguez Milagros. Hygiene of removable prostheses in patients attended at the San Gregorio University of Portoviejo, Ecuador 2019. Rev. inf. cient. [Internet]. 2020 Jun [cited 2024 Mar 21]; 99(3): 217-224. Available from: http://scielo.sld.cu/scielo.php?script=sci_arttext&pid=S1028-99332020000300217&lng=en.

44- Ramos Lorenzo Mavel, Hernández Miranda Leinad, Castellanos Curbelo Alienne. Care and conservation of acrylic prostheses in geriatric patients at the Clínica Estomatológica Puentes Grandes.Rev Eug Esp [Internet]. 2019Dec [cited 2024 Mar 22]; 13(2): 53-61. Available from: http://scielo.senescyt.gob.ec/scielo.php?script=sci_arttext&pid=S2661-67422019000200053&lng=en. https://doi.org/10.37135/ee.004.7.06

45- Guzmán-Gallardo H, Ubilla-Mazzini W, Suarez-Palacios JC. Cleft Epulis: its effects on the treatment of the upper total edentulous patient: Epulis Fisurado: sus afectaciones en el tratamiento de el paciente edéntulo total superior: Cleft Epulis: its effects on the treatment of the upper total edentulous patient. EOUG [Internet]. July 4, 2023 [cited March 18, 2024];6(2):44-50. Available from: https://revistas.ug.edu.ec/index.php/eoug/article/view/2177

46- Morgado LY, Reyes RDE, Oliva VME, et al. Methodology of the oral complex examination for stomatology students. April 16. 2015[cited 2024 Feb 13];54 (258):74-82.Available from : https://www.medigraphic.com/cgi-bin/new/resumen.cgi?IDARTICULO=61579

47- Nápoles González Isidro de Jesús, Nápoles Salas Ana María. Social need of stomatological care for the elderly with dysmobility. Rev Hum Med [Internet]. 2021 Apr [cited 2024 Mar 24] ; 21(1): 209-223. Available from:

http://scielo.sld.cu/scielo.php?script=sci_arttext&pid=S1727-81202021000100209&lng=en
48- Yero-Mier IM, Pérez-García LM, Fernández-Serrano JM. Paraprosthetic injuries in geriatric patients with removable prostheses. Rev Inf Cient [Internet]. 2021 [cited day month year]; 100(4):e3462. Available from: http://www.revinfcientifica.sld.cu/index.php/ric/article/view/3462
49- Rodríguez Baquero IL, Forero Escobar D, Díaz Y, Mendoza L. Prevalence of oral lesions associated with removable dental prostheses in Villavicencio. Universidad Cooperativa de Colombia [Internet].2020 [cited 2024 Mar 20] [approx 11] [approx 11]available at: https://repository.ucc.edu.co/bitstreams/97dd7324-1757-42fa-9370-83f5d516135d/download
50- Martínez González RI. Perception of dentists in the city of Concepción on oral mucosal lesions related to removable partial dentures in 2019:
Perception of dentists in the city of Concepción on lesions in the oral mucosa linked to removable partial dentures in 2019. OSS FOUNC [Internet]. July 1, 2021 [cited 2024 March 24];2(1):40-6. Available from: https://revistas.unc.edu.py/index.php/founc/article/view/21
51- Rodríguez-Pimienta EM, Yero-Mier IM, Pérez-Garcia LM, de Castro-Yero JL, Marín-Montero. I, García-Luis Y. Subprosthetic stomatitis in patients with removable prostheses at the Camilo Cienfuegos military school. Sancti Spíritus. Rev Ciencias Médicas [Internet]. 2022 [cited: 2024 Mar 20]; 26(1): e5055. Available from: http://revcmpinar.sld.cu/index.php/publicaciones/article/view/5055
52- Cruz-Sixto D, Palacios-Sixto A, Perdomo-Acosta A, González-Camejo D, Arencibia- García E. Causal factors in the appearance of oral lesions in older adults. Universidad Médica Pinareña [journal on the Internet]. 2020 [cited 17 Mar 2024]; 16 (2) Available from:

https://revgaleno.sld.cu/index.php/ump/article/view/422
53- Eugen R, Scrieciu M, Mercut V, Popescu S, Andrei O, Pitru A, et al. Oral mucosa associated with wearing removable acrylic denture. Rev. Cur Health Sci Jornual [Internet]. 2020 [cited 2024 Mar 20];46(4):344-351. Available from https://www.ncbi.nlm.nih.gov/pmc/articles/PMC7948026/
54- García Rodríguez B, Rodríguez Cuellar Y, GonzálezCardona Y. Subprosthetic stomatitis in total and partial edentulous patients. Rev. Latinoamericana de Hipertensión [Internet].2022[cited 2024 Mar 19];17(4):289-293.Available from: http://saber.ucv.ve/ojs/index.php/rev_lh/article/view/25640
55- Salazar Gamez JE.Presencia de lesiones bucales en adultos mayores portadores de prótesis dental que acuden al hospital maría auxiliadora, Lima 2023 [Thesis] aprox 98.Available in: https://hdl.handle.net/20.500.12692/133144
56- González Feria R k.Characterization of oral lesions in removable prosthesis wearers. Julio Antonio Mella University Teaching Polyclinic. Holguín. 2022. [Thesis] approx 57 Available at: https://tesis.hlg.sld.cu/index.php?P=DownloadFile&Id=2759
57- Arias Fernández C, Ramírez Santiago A C, Meza García .Prevalence and Risk Factors of Oral Mucosal Lesions in the Population of Oaxaca de Juárez .Revista Espacio Universitario. 15 (39), 45, 2020 [cited2024Mar 19]. Disponible en:https://scholar.google.es/scholar?as_ylo=2020&q=relaci%C3%B3n+entre+factores+de+riesgo+y+lesiones+de+la+mucosa+oral+&hl=es&as_sdt=0,5#d=gs_qabs&t=171614537 4735&u=%23p%3DOC7GQJMEKV0J

ANNEXES

ANNEX 1. QUESTIONNAIRE FOR OLDER ADULT PATIENTS

Objective: To find out what information the patients in the sample have about oral conditions associated with the use of dental prostheses and oral hygiene.
Questionnaire of questions:

1. How many times a day do you clean or brush your prosthesis?

Once 2 times 3 times 4 times

2. How long have you been wearing dentures? --

Up to 5

6-10 years

11-15 years

16- 20more than 20

3. Is the prosthesis removed to sleep?
Yes No
4. Do you feel that the prosthesis falls off or moves when eating or talking? Yes No
5. Do you smoke?
No Always Occasionally

ANNEX 2. DATA COLLECTION FORM

Objective: To record information related to the characteristics of oral lesions.

1. General data:

Age: 60-69 years old 70-79 years old 80 years and over Sex: F M

2. Classification of the injury:

✓ Subprosthetic stomatitis

Present Not present

✓ Traumatic ulcers

Present Not present

✓ Epulis fissured

Present Not present

✓ Leukoplakia

Present Not present

✓ Erythroplasia

Present Not present

3. Daily **Smoking** Occasionally No smoking

4. Type of prosthesis Total

Upper Lower **Partial** Upper Inferior

5. Type of prosthesis material:

Acrylic Metal Mixed

6. Time of use of the prosthesis.

Up to 5 years old 6 to 10 years

11 to 20 years old Over 20 years old

7. Frequency of use of the prosthesis.

Correct. Incorrect .

8. Hygiene of the prosthesis.

Yes No

9. Condition of the prosthesis.

Good Fair Bad

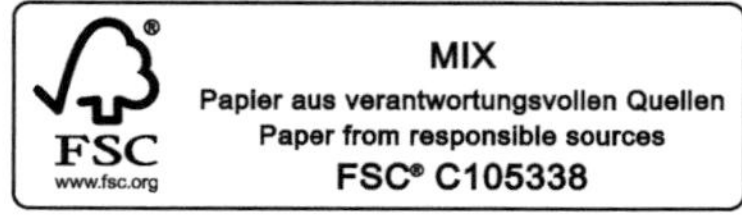

Printed by Books on Demand GmbH, Norderstedt / Germany